TIGHT HIP FLEXORS

Simple Workout Principle in Maintaining Flexibility, To Relieve, and Cure You of Pain in Less Than 5 Minutes

Charles Belcher

TABLE OF CONTENT

CHAPTER ONE

WHAT DOES HIP FLEXO MEAN

First, help your clients recognize what the hip flexors are, what they do, and how you understand once they're tight. The time period hip flexors refer to a group of muscle tissues in and across the hips that assist pass the legs and the trunk together, as when you lifting your leg in an upper direction, while bending at the hip.

The Hip Flexor Muscle organization

The hip flexor consists of:

The iliopsoas, which is virtually two muscles, the psoas, and the iliacus,

The tensor fasciae latae,

The rectus femoris,

And the Sartorius

The muscular tissues produce flexion through their movement and tightening of the muscle mass that permits flexing of the hip joint. Collectively, they help in stabilizing the backbone.

Strengthening the core is vital to supporting the hip flexors, however, are taking a seat-united state the nice manner to work your abs?

We have the answer right here.

CHAPTER TWO

GREAT STRETCHES FOR TIGHT HIP FLEXO

Your hip flexors are a collection of muscle groups close to the pinnacle of your thighs that are key players in moving your decrease body. They can help you to walk, kick, bend, and swivel your hips. However in case your muscles are too tight or if you make a surprising motion, your hip flexors can stretch or tear.

A hip flexor pressure can be mildly uncomfortable or so severe which you have trouble strolling and feature muscle spasms and lot of pain.

Ordinary stretches can assist preserve your hip flexors free and prevent injuries.

Standing Stretch

Stand with your toes hip-width apart and ft ahead.

Bend your right knee, and convey your right heel up toward your butt.

Keep your proper foot with the proper hand, and lightly pull to point your knee in the direction of the floor. You may maintain directly to a counter or chair along with your left hand for balance.

Hold for 30 seconds. Repeat for your different leg.

Active Stretch

Stand to your left foot with the ft barely turned inward. put your right foot on the seat of a chair in the front of you.

Preserve your palms directly out in the front of you at chest degree.

Slowly increase your arms instantly up as you squeeze your butt and lightly push your pelvis ahead. That will straighten your left leg and deepen the bend for your proper knee. You'll experience the stretch within the front of your left hip.

Go back to the beginning position and repeat on the other leg.

Kneeling Stretch

Kneel along with your left knee at the ground and your proper leg at a ninety-degree attitude in the front of you.

Placed your hands on your right knee and maintain you're returned directly.

Retaining your left knee pressed to the floor, lean forward into your proper hip while squeezing the muscle tissue in your left buttocks.

Preserve for 30 seconds. Repeat on the opposite facet.

CHAPTER THREE

SIGNS TO SHOW ONE HAVE TIGHT HIP FLEXO

The obvious sign, of the route, is that these muscle tissues just experience tight. You try to stretch them and that they don't circulate a whole lot. But there are other signs and symptoms too. Tight hip flexor muscle groups can affect several other regions of your body, so you might have:

Tightness or an ache in your lower returned, mainly while status.

Poor posture and problem status up straight.

Neck tightness and pain

Ache in the glutes.

You could additionally do a test to evaluate tightness. Lying to your back on a table or bench, pull one knee up in the direction of your chest and hold it there. Permit the opposite leg to loosen up down over the brink of the desk. It facilitates here to have a person preserve that leg for you so you can do it slowly.

If your hip flexors are high-quality you must be capable of completely extend the thigh so it's parallel to the floor and bend the knee to 90 tiers without the thigh rising up. Any problem with those moves suggests tight hip flexor muscular tissues.

CHAPTER FOUR

CAUSES OF TIGHT HIP FLEXO

For most people, the biggest cause of tightness is what we do all day lengthy: sitting for too lengthy is a major perpetrator in tightening the hip flexors. When you sit all day at a desk, the iliopsoas, especially, shortens, making the flexors tight.

A few athletes are also extra prone to tightness. Runners use the hip flexors, particularly the iliopsoas, to lift the leg up with each stride. This repeated shortening of the muscle isn't compensated for by means of a lengthening motion. Runners regularly turn out to be with tight hip flexors because of this.

Having a susceptible center can also be a difficulty that contributes to tight hip flexors. Due to the fact these muscle groups are linked to and stabilize the spine, they often take over whilst the core isn't always sturdy. This could result in tightening and pain.

CHAPTER FIVE

STRETCHES AND EXERCISES TO LOOSEN UP AND STRENGTHEN TIGHT HIP FLEXOS

Having tight hip flexors can motive accidents, pain, and restrained mobility, so it's well worth taking a couple of minutes in keeping with the day to stretch them out when you have tightness. Right here are some stretches to try, for you or your clients:

Foam roll: A foam curler can be useful in stretching and loosening hip muscle mass. Get right into a forearm plank function on the floor with the roller underneath the front of one hip. Permit the opposite leg to stay out to the facet, of the curler. Roll up and down for approximately 30 seconds, specializing in factors that sense especially tight.

Pigeon pose: Borrow this pass from yoga to stretch out the flexors. On your arms and knees, pull the proper knee forward. Bend it beneath your chest and stretch out the left leg in the back of you. Lay down on the pinnacle of your bent knee as plenty as you may. With tight muscle groups, it could make the effort before you could do that absolutely, so take it slowly.

Butterfly stretch: Take a seat on the ground with the bottoms of your ft pressed together. Allow the knees to fall outward to stretch the hips. For a further stretch, gently push down to your knees.

Low lunge: Carry out a deep lunge with the right leg forward. Gently let the left knee resting on the ground and straighten that leg a lot as viable. Put your fingers flat on every aspect of the right foot, then improve the left arm up above your head and lean to the right. Maintain some seconds and repeat on the other facet.

Moves that support the hip muscle tissues, the glutes, and the center will all be beneficial in preventing tightness in the hip flexors in addition to accidents. Those movements can enhance strength and offer a terrific stretch at an equal time:

Glute bridges: This pass wills paintings your hips, middle, and glutes. Mendacity to your again with knees bent, carry the hips up as excessive as viable, and squeeze the glutes. To make it greater hard, pass one leg over the other knee and lift one side at a time.

Unmarried-leg squat: To truly focus in vicinity at a time, attempt an unmarried leg skating squat. lower into an ordinary squat and raise one leg up and returned as you upward push lower back as much as a status role. Stretch the other leg out straight to prolong hip flexors at the same time as additionally running the glutes.

Mountain climbers: In plank position on your hands, exchange bringing each knee ahead, towards your chest. You may use sliders for this and do it both fast and sluggish to work each hip and abs.

Learn extra about the flexible, effective squat, and what correct form without a doubt looks as if in this ISSA blog post.

Hip flexor tightness may be a real ache, but working certain muscle mass and doing the right stretches provide easy fixes. Help your customers be more aware of their hips and diagnose any issues so you can accurately them before they go through injuries.

CHAPTER SIX

WHAT MAKES UP THE HIP JOINT

Which will begin enhancing the mobility of your hips and the way they move, you have to realize what makes up this vital frame element

The hip is a ball-and-socket synovial joint (fancy call for two bones joined together with fluid that allows easy movements) that permits the best amount of range of motion as compared to any joint inside the body besides the shoulder. It includes the femur (head of the femur makes the ball) and the acetabulum of the pelvis (that is the socket). Surrounding this joint is a massive quantity of muscular tissues, ligaments, and cartilage that have attachments to the hip.

As physical therapists, we're taught to continually check the regions above and below the goal joint. This gives you a higher photo and evaluation of what you're dealing with.

Above your hips, you have your center. Believe it or now not, so that you can flow the pelvis successfully, you need to know the way to stabilize the spine. The abdominals will assist you to do that. The middle acts like a corset such as the transverse abdominals, rectus abdominals, and inner and outside oblique's. When activated, will hold the entirety together tightly and hold the whole thing stabilized.

Underneath your hips, you've got all of the essential muscle tissue with attachments to the legs that assist in liberating up the hips. You have predominant muscle organizations along with the quadriceps, iliopsoas, adductors, hamstrings, and glutes. placed in the front of your hip you have your hip flexors, those muscle tissue frequently get tight and stiff when sitting for long intervals of time. Inside the returned you have your glutes and hamstrings; those are activated normally at some point of walking and the usage of the stairs. On the inside of your leg are your adductors; these muscular tissues are responsible for bringing your legs closer to your frame's centerline (the line that divides your frame into left and right). Ultimately, at the outside of your legs are your abductors, used anytime you move your legs far from the centerline. These muscle tissues all play a large function in the lower body motion in each day's tasks.

CHAPTER SEVEN

DIET DESIGNED FOR HEALTHY HIPS

It is less difficult to guard our hips if we take steps to maintain them strong whilst we are more youthful.

As we age, the muscle tissues helping our hip and leg movement lose electricity. At the same time, bone density and electricity decline. As bones become extra fragile, the hazard of hip fracture increases. Women are specifically at hazard; half of all women age 50 and older will fracture or wreck a bone due to osteoporosis.

Whilst the injured bone is a hip bone, the results are especially severe. Half of those who go through a hip fracture don't regain complete function. One region of them loses their independence, requiring nursing domestic care. Hip fractures are existence-threatening. One out of each 5 folks who enjoy a hip fracture dies within 12 months of the damage.

The good news is that there are a number of proactive steps you may take now to lessen your fracture threat. Everyday exercising, awareness around fall dangers, monitoring bone density, and keeping off smoking are all important.

you can additionally help to lessen your fracture chance by means of cultivating a bone-healthful weight-reduction plan with an emphasis on calcium and diet D. properly sources of calcium and diet D encompass the following:

Low-fat dairy merchandise like milk, yogurt, and cheese

Fortified ingredients include breakfast cereal and orange juice.

Leafy veggies like spinach are also top; however, you'll need to eat a lot extra of them to equal the calcium advantages of dairy meals.

Fatty fish is a good source of vitamin D, so preserve salmon on the menu often.

Calcium fuels an array of frame functions. Whilst there isn't sufficient calcium for your food regimen, your body will take it from your bones. Girls over 50 want 1, 2 hundred mg of calcium a day. An excessive amount of calcium, however, will make an awesome element better. In case you devour greater than 2,000 mg an afternoon, your threat of developing kidney stones will increase.

Vitamin D is the agent that allows your frame to take in the calcium you consume. You want between 800 and 1,000 IUs of vitamin D every day, but don't late it. Extra than 4,000 IUs each day can cause kidney and cardiovascular troubles.

THE END

9 798592 056802